Pain Relief

Essential Oils and Herbal Remedies

Table of Contents

Introduction

I would first like to thank you and congratulate you on downloading *"Essential Oils: Herbal Remedies for Pain Relief."* Choosing to learn more about healthy medicinal options is a good step on your part. I am sure that you will be more than pleased with the results that you will gain from using this collection of herbal remedies.

Many people will often put taking care of their health off, always rushing back and forth from one meeting to the next. Never stopping long enough to put some time and effort in to looking after their health. This is even more prevalent in today's fast paced world, with high levels of all kinds of stressors in people's daily lives. These are great reasons why you should make it must do to put some time and effort into caring for your mental and physical health.

You do not have to have expensive health treatments that are costly and take up too much time. You can make use of the wonderful selection of essential oils that can help you to achieve that balance you are seeking without take large sums of money and time to accomplish your goals.

Using home remedies such as the collection in this book can help you to avoid suffering pain and stress in a natural and therapeutic way. Essential oils have been used by mankind for literally centuries in treating ailments and helping us to relax and physically feel better. You can use natural home remedies to treat your ailments without having to resort to expensive pharmaceutical synthetic drugs. In this book I offer you knowledge about what essential oils are and their uses along with a collection of great remedies that will have you feeling like your old self in no time!

Chapter 1. What Are Essential Oils?

Essential oils are basically different elements of
plants that can be used in different ways in order
to help us to heal. One part of the plant is the
aroma, another part is the oils of the plants. The
oils extracted from medicinal plants are known to
have certain health benefits. They are great for
someone that is looking for relieve of ailments
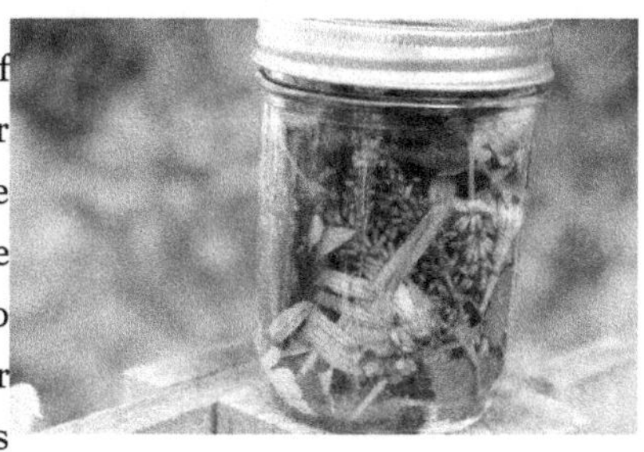
without resorting to pharmaceutical products, but choosing essential oils from nature
instead.

The oils themselves are extracted from parts of the plants such as the flowers, leaves and
berries. One of my own personal favourites of these plants is the lavender plant. It has
such a great aroma. The lavender essential oil is often used to help people gain a sense
of well-being and calmness.

There are different ways that the essential oils can be extracted from the plants.
Methods such as cold pressing, steam distillation are included in these processes. A true
essential oil will only contain what was taken from the plant itself. It will have a thick
consistency, but rarely is it sticky.

There are many manufacturers of these essential oils that will add to them artificial
ingredients in an attempt to supposedly "enhance" the natural product that mother
nature has offered to us. These results are not as effective as the pure essential oils.
They can often be laced with chemicals that are added to make the oil look and smell
more acceptable.

Essential oils contain very potent ingredients from nature. In a pure essential oil you
can expect it to have contents that will include aromatic properties such as in the case of
lavender, as well as offering therapeutic ingredients. Many essential oils offer more

than one benefit. Take for example eucalyptus essential oil is very good in helping to treat breathing problems from a cough. It also has agents within it that will help the healing process of tired muscles.

Common Sources of Essential Oils

Essential oils that are taken from plants and used in their pureness are used in treating many different ailments. Some of the common plants used for their beneficial properties are sage, basil, eucalyptus, bergamot, rose, lavender, clary, lemon balm. Frankincense, spearmint, marjoram, geranium, Vetiver, peppermint, clove, juniper and ylang ylang.

 Imagine you are peeling an orange, think of the wonderful aroma that is released from the zest of the orange during the peeling process this will help you to better understand what essential oils are.

The zest from peel is cold pressed to produce the oils that people recognize as essential oils. Essential oils due to being non-sticky fluids are mixed with "carrier-oils" such as almond oil, olive oil, carrot seed oil, coconut oil, and sesame oil. You should always use pure essential oils.

As you can imagine it takes a lot of plants and plant parts to make a small amount of the precious pure essential oils. They can seem expensive, but when you compare them to the high costs of pharmaceutical drugs they are actually fairly reasonable in price. Especially when you consider that they are natural pure products unlike the chemical filled commercial pharmaceutical products that come with side effects.

Essential oils can also be produced from seeds. The cardamom seed is a very powerful seed used in producing essential oils. This particular seed is often used in Indian cuisine. The oil format of the seed can be very beneficial for digestion, and also good in helping people to breathe better. The wood from the tree can also be used to produce essential oils. The smell of cedar wood for example is known to be beneficial for many common ailments.

Essential oils are produced from nature. That is the most simple way to describe them. The methods used in extracting the oils are many different forms that are quite complex.

Origin of Essential Oils

The history of essential oils being used in healing dates back thousands of years back in human history. There has been evidence of the recorded use of healing oils dating back to early Egyptian times.

Aromatherapy is a form of therapy that uses the aroma of essential oils that may be diffused into the air surrounding us to offer us comfort and a sense of well-being. Mankind has been using the healing benefits of the essential oils for thousands of years—using nothing more than the pure essential oils offered to us by mother nature.

Essential Oils can Cure and Prevent Ailments

Most of us are familiar with the famous adage "prevention is better than the cure." When you use essential oils they will not only cure ailments, but prevent them from recurring. Essential oils have immunity boosting powers, unlike commercial medicines, this will help to prevent diseases.

You can make essential oils as part of your daily life even when you are not ill, to help keep your body healthy without side-effects. How will this help you? There are certain aromas that help humans to feel well. Just imagine you are smelling a fresh boutique of roses, or coriander, sage. Feel how mint can help your body to breath with ease again. It may not be a particular illness that is causing symptoms it could be down to bad habits such as smoking. Smoking will cause your lungs and bronchial passages to be blocked and essential oils can put that right and make the user feel the advantages almost immediately.

Think of walking into a room that you are greeted with a pleasant odor and how that made you feel. Common aromas that are known to help the human wellbeing are aromas such as lime, lemongrass, and marjoram. Each of these essential oils will make your body feel stimulated and at peace.

When the essential oils are released there are so many aspects of health that they can touch, from aiding in the healing of skin to helping your hair look healthy and shiny. When essential oils release their goodness you will instantly feel the positive benefits that are derived from them.

Using the essential oil Ylang Ylang can help in achieving balance in the hormones. Wild Orange essential oil is great at helping to purify the skin and boost the immunity system. When it comes to the benefits of essential oils it is difficult to list all of them. The reason being is that nature has a special way of producing results from unexpected places and benefits of one essential oil can cover so many aspects in life.

Take the example of wild orange essential oil, it can be used for dual or even triple purpose. It can be used to help boost the immunity system, skin and also to help protect the body from seasonal changes in the atmosphere and weather conditions. This essential oil can help to refresh the mind and leave you feeling invigorated, so you don't need to limit your use of essential oils to only when you are ill.

Use essential oils as a prevention that you can incorporate into your life. Adding essential oils into your life will help you to avoid illnesses so that you do not have to deal with the pressure of dealing with them.

It is definitely a wiser choice to choose prevention rather than waiting to you are ill and need to seek a cure. Why put your body through undo stress when you do not have to.

Chapter 2. Why Essential Oils Are a Good Choice of Medicine

Essential oils are a good choice in medicine for many different reasons. One of the main and important reasons that they are a good choice of medical treatment is that they do not harm the human body. They also do not come with the harmful side effects that modern medicines do. All you need to do is to look at pharmaceutical medications and look at the list of "secondary side effects" that accompany them, these can run on and on. People can react to the same 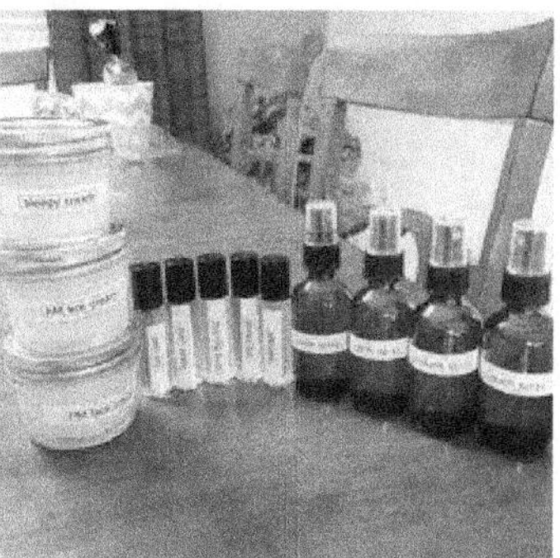 medications differently. Even though the pharmaceutical medications have been tested as safe by the FDA, they will still come with a string of secondary side effects as a consequence of taking the synthetic medication.

Good Value in Essential Oils

When you invest into purchasing a set of essential oils you are going to have a medical cabinet right in your home at all times, especially when needed. When you become used to using essential oils as a form of treatment for many common ailments you will have to visit the doctor less and less. You will also not have to fill out expensive prescriptions anymore or at least not as often as you once did before you began to use essential oils.

Make sure and check the bottles of essential oils to make sure that no other ingredients have been added to them and that they are indeed pure essential oils. There is cheaper forms of essential oils, these are cheaper grades of oil that have been mixed with other ingredients. Get the best which is pure essential oils when using them for medicinal purposes.

No Side Effects

Your pure essential oils come from herbal and natural sources that are derived from medicinal plants. When using these essential oils holistically and under proper supervision, no harm will come to you. Compared to synthetic pharmaceutical drugs, pure essential oils have basically zero harmful side effects. Even using essential oils for a prolonged period of time will not cause you harm unlike pharmaceutical drugs.

Even though essential oils do not have any side effects, it is essential to check whether you are allergic to an oil before you use it. You should always take allergies into account when using any product to help with health issues. If you have allergies to a natural element then it is very possible that you will also be allergic to any oils associated with that natural element. With that being said you should make sure to avoid using that particular type of oil. However, there is many other essential oils that I am sure you will benefit from by adding them to your health regime.

Market Availability

Essential oils are readily available unlike prescription medications, either over the counter or through an internet website. You can also find essential oils in a variety of stores such as health food stores. You do not need to have a prescription to purchase essential oils. You may even decide to grow your own medicinal garden. This is one of the main reasons that essential oils are becoming one of the most popular alternative medicines—in that you can easily begin to grow your own supply of medicinal plants that you can extract the oils from.

Using Essential Oils to Treat Chronic Illnesses

There are many chronic diseases such as arthritis, as well as severe back pains and aches that often will require prolonged use of drugs. It is not advised to use modern drugs for a prolonged period, as these drugs may cause harmful side effects. If you are someone suffering from arthritis for example, you may have been prescribed anti-inflammatory drugs to reduce inflammation. However, accompanying these drugs could be unwanted side effects, and often you will be prescribed more drugs to counter those side effects. It becomes a vicious circle and one that chronically ill people find very hard to cope with. Using good holistic medicines for these chronic illnesses won't cause harm even after prolonged use. Essential oils are thus better to use to treat these ailments. These disorders often respond very well to being treated with essential oils.

Safety

Many modern day drugs use components that are derived from natural ingredients like plant sources. There are many drugs that contain essential oil extracts. So why not choose the totally natural choice and go with just the essential oils instead of risking serious side-effects with man-made modern drugs. Essential oils have been used for thousands of years throughout the world, many different cultures use them in their medicinal and culinary needs. Herbal remedies have been used throughout human history, with ancient remedies passed down from generation to generation, these can be considered a safe alternative to modern day drugs.

Multiple Benefits

Essential oils do not pin point an exact disease or disorder unlike modern medicines. Often a user of essential oil remedies can take it for one ailment and they may hone in on other ailments the user may be suffering from as well. So essential oils basically have multiple benefits and thus are much better then commercial medications that are prescribed for a specific ailment. You could for example find that your breathing has improved as a side consequence of using essential oil remedy for perhaps digestive problems. So, it ends up that the benefits can have an enormous impact by helping to improve your health in numerous ways all at once. Essential oils offer many essential nutrients which are required by the human body, which come from natural sources with no side effects.

Chapter 3. Common Essential Oils & Their Uses

Peppermint Essential Oil

When it comes to breathing problems peppermint essential oil is a typical favorite to use. Peppermint essential oil is also good at treating problems with the digestive system. This is a great essential oil that is great for daily family life.

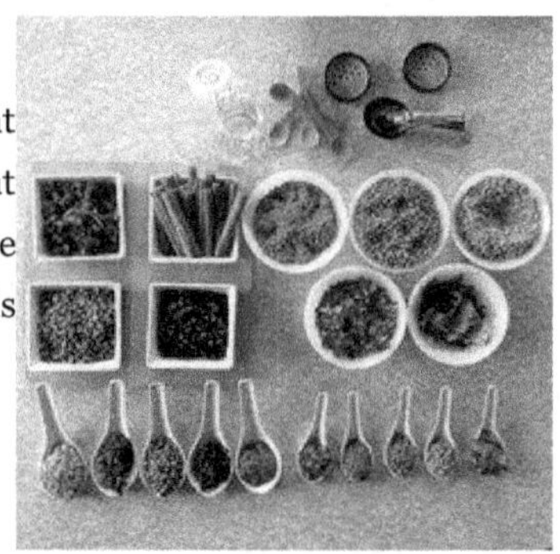

Wild Orange Essential Oil

The wonderful zesty aroma of wild orange essential oil helps with so many things. You may remember as a child your mother asking you to eat an orange to get your vitamin C. The oils from wild orange essential oil will help to ward of colds, they also will protect you from environmental changes and help your immune system to stay energized and alert.

Lavender Essential Oil

Most of us love the smell of lavender for good reason. The aroma of lavender is a feel good aroma which helps us to calm down. It is also good in treating headaches and skin irritations. This is a very popular choice of essential oil.

Fennel Essential Oil

Fennel is often used by women dealing with menstrual cramps. It is also good at helping the lymphatic system to stay healthy. It is most used as a remedy for digestion related issues such as anorexia, nausea, constipation, flatulence, hiccups and vomiting. It can also be used in the treatment of obesity, it helps to promote the feeling of being full and has a diuretic effect which disperses cellulite.

Eucalyptus Essential Oil

Eucalyptus is a common flavor used in cough sweets. Eucalyptus essential oil is a natural coolant. It offers a cooling and deodorizing effect on the human body in treating ailments such as malaria, fevers and migraine. It is also effective in the treatment of coughs, asthma, sinusitis, and throat infections. It contains anti-inflammatory properties, soothing inflammation and easing mucus, and also helping in eliminating stuffiness due to hay fever and colds. It can also be used as a warming oil for muscular pains and sprains or even for poor circulation. Eucalyptus essential oil also works very well on cuts, burns, blisters, wounds and other skin conditions. You can use eucalyptus essential oil to gain some relief when suffering from measles, chicken pox or the flu.

Basil Essential Oil

Basil like many plants mentioned are often found in herb gardens. Basil essential oil is good to use to help alleviate sore muscles, helps to calm, it works well especially after a sporting event. It works good in treating breathing problems as well, and will also help to keep your skin cool in the hot summer months.

Clove Essential Oil

Clove essential oil is really good to use in keeping your gums and teeth healthy. Cloves are good at helping the heart stay healthy, they act as an antioxidant.

Thyme Essential Oil

Thyme is great at helping to ward off effects from the winter or changing seasons, it helps to cleanse your skin, while it wards off seasonal changes. It will also strengthen nerves, and will help improve your memory and concentration. Thyme will also help to relieve depression, exhaustion and fatigue.

Thyme is great to use in treating whooping cough, sinusitis, asthma, flu and colds. It also helps to boost the immune system and acts as a urinary antiseptic. It also offers a warming effect that can help with poor circulation and help with injuries such as sprains. Thyme is also known to help treat obesity and cellulite.

Sandalwood Essential Oil

Sandalwood oil is commonly used in the Indian subcontinent. The oil is extracted from the wood of the sandalwood tree. It is considered holy in India and is quite costly. It is predominantly used in India along with being used often in Yoga related schools of health. It helps to calm the mind. It is also good at helping to keep balance of emotions. This oil works great if you are looking to create a calm atmosphere so perhaps you can meditate.

Rosemary Essential Oil

Rosemary essential oil is very useful in treating digestive problems. The oil also gives off an aroma that is useful as an anti-inflammatory. It can be applied to areas of strained muscles by a topical cream, or during a massage treatment.

Tea Tree Essential Oil

Tea tree essential oil is one of the most potent and important essential oils. It offers a light spicy fragrance, extracted from Melaleuca alternifolia. It will help to ensure the health of your immune system. Tea tree oil is becoming more widely used within the cosmetic industry for its many benefits. It helps to increase the body's immunity thus helps ward off diseases and infections.

Tea tree essential oil can help with cold sores, fever, influenza, glandular fever, whooping cough, sinusitis, tuberculosis, and bronchial congestion. It is also beneficial in treating vaginal thrush and warts and other genital infections. It contains anti-inflammatory properties and helps treat burns, acne, greasy skin herpes, blemishes, sunburns and infected wounds.

Nutmeg Essential Oil

Nutmeg essential oil is often used to fight off muscle pain and inflammation through the use of aromatherapy. It also offers a wonderful invigorating and stimulating effect on the mind as well. The therapeutic properties of nutmeg essential oil range from analgesic to anti-rheumatic, antiseptic, laxative, digestive, antispasmodic, carminative, stimulant and tonic.

It is also effective in stimulating the heart and helps with circulation, makes the mind more active. It works great for people that suffer from fainting spells. It helps to strengthen the digestive tract. It can also help to relieve diarrhea, chronic vomiting, nausea. It helps give you a healthy appetite while avoiding constipation, it also acts like a tonic for the reproductive system, fighting off frigidity and impotence.

Pine Essential Oil

Pine essential oil has many benefits with its therapeutic properties, such as antimicrobial, antiviral, antiseptic, bactericidal, diuretic, deodorant, hypertensive, expectorant, insecticidal, restorative as well as a stimulant.

It works well at providing relief of fatigue, can be used in vapor therapy to provide one with an invigorating effect. It treats sexual, mental and physical fatigue effectively. It can also be used in treating cuts and sores. It helps to treat rheumatism due to its warming effects. It can be also used in treating asthma, muscular aches and pains, laryngitis, flu and colds. You can also use it to get rid of scabies and lice. It also acts like a cleanser for your kidneys helping to prevent urinary infections.

Jasmine Essential Oil

Jasmine essential oil works well in treating depression and helps to lift the spirits and enables confidence. It can also assist with sexual problems, soothe coughs and will enhance the elasticity in your skin, while lessen the appearance of stretch marks.

The wonderful properties of jasmine essential oil help to work as an anti-depressant, antiseptic, sedative, cicatrisant, expectorant, galactagogue, parturient, calming and uterine. It will help you retain the feeling of contentment, happiness and confidence, while at the same time revitalizing your body. It is good to use during post-natal depression and also helps to get the breast milk flowing. It is also good for aiding with sexual issues such as impotency, frigidity, and premature ejaculation. Jasmine can also help to relieve laryngitis and coughs. It offers a nice cooling effect to the skin. It works wonders for dry skin and reducing skin scars.

Frankincense Essential Oil

Frankincense essential oil has a cooling effect on the brain through aromatherapy. It helps to make internal peace, while it soothes the respiratory, urinary tracts, and pains that are related to stiffness and muscular pains and aches. It will help to make your skin feel revived. It has therapeutic properties that allow it to work as an astringent, germicide, digestive, expectorant, calming tonic, carminative, uterine, and vulnerary.

Frankincense works great at helping to calm, works great during meditation. It helps to surpress anxiety. It helps to clear the lungs and help with shortness of breath, asthma, bronchitis, laryngitis hacks and colds. It helps to alleviate menstrual cramps. It is also effective on wounds, sores and scars.

Cinnamon Essential Oil

Cinnamon essential oil is often used in aromatherapy with its musky, warm and spicy fragrance. Some of the therapeutic properties for it are an antiseptic, cardiac, analgesic, aphrodisiac, antibiotic, tonic, stimulant and vermifuge. It can help to get rid of flu and colds and will help to reduce depression and weakness. It can be used to help treat infected respiratory tracts. It also can help in treating arthritis, rheumatism and other general aches and pains.

Camphor Essential Oil

This is a very valuable essential oil when it comes to remedying colds. You can use it as part of a vapor therapy to clear lungs, to dispel apathy, and calm nervous depression. It also offers a number of skin benefits that you could use in daily beauty regime. The therapeutic benefits it offers are of antiseptic, cardiac, diuretic, analgesic, febrifuge, stimulant and antidepressant. It is also a great aide in the treatment of inflammation, acne, muscular aches, colds, fevers, rheumatism, depression, flu and other infectious diseases. When it comes to aromatherapy camphor oil should be avoided, owing to its toxic properties. It is best to use it in a vapor therapy, or even in compresses.

Black Pepper Essential Oil

The black pepper essential oil is spicy and helps induce warmth in the body, thus proving it to be a great remedy for colds. It is also good to use for treating joint aches and sore muscles. It also helps with circulation, rheumatoid arthritis, and bruising. It is most commonly used in the treatment of muscular aches, nerve tonic, for fevers, pain relief, helping to stimulate the appetite, enables peristalsis, helping to facilitate proper digestion. If you overuse this essential oil it could lead to irritation of the skin, or over stimulation of the kidneys. The overall therapeutic properties of black pepper essential oil are diuretic, digestive, antispasmodic, laxative, analgesic, and antiseptic in nature.

Chapter 4. Suggested Recipes for Various Ailments

1. Headache Mixture

Ingredients:

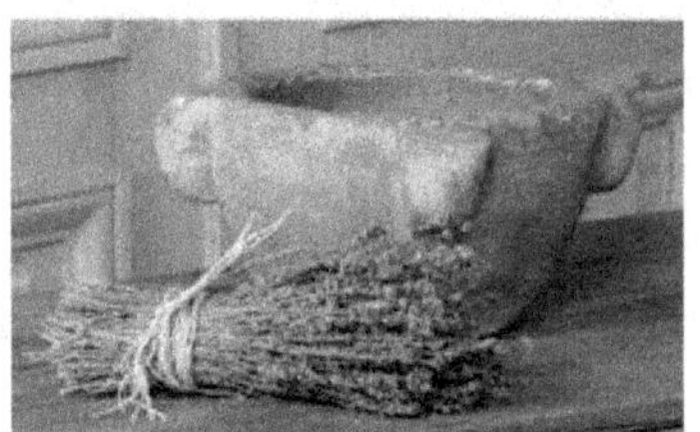

- 7 drops of rosemary essential oil

- 15 drops of lavender essential oil

- 80ml of almond oil

- 7 drops of basil essential oil

Directions:

In a small dark, glass vial add in the ingredients. Roll the vial around in the palm of your hand to mix oils together. Inhale the oils for a minute to gain the stress relief effect. You can also use it as a balm as well, make sure to mix it with at least a tablespoon of carrier oil.

2. Lift Up Your Spirits

The ingredients in this recipe are to help lift up your spirits by relieving tension and stress.

Ingredients:

- 2 drops of Wild Orange essential oil

- 4 drops of peppermint essential oil

Directions:

Apply wild orange essential oil and wrists and feet and layer with peppermint essential oil. Add a drop of peppermint on back of neck to help with cooling.

3. Feel Good

This mix will offer you a feel good factor that will help to relieve stress at the same time.

Ingredients:

- 4 drops of cedarwood essential oil

- 3 drops of lavender essential oil

- 3 drops of geranium essential oil

Directions:

Add all of the ingredients into a small dark vial. Roll the vial around in your palm to mix oils. Inhale the oils for a minute or so. You can add at least a tablespoon of carrier oil and make a balm.

4.   Lemon & Cedarwood Mixture

This mix of essential oils is very therapeutic for treating colds, flu and stuffed up noses.

Ingredients:

- 2 drops of lemon essential oil

- 2 drops of cedarwood essential oil

- 2 drops of lavender essential oil

Directions:

Add all of the ingredients into a small dark vial. Roll the vial around in your palm to mix oils. Inhale the oils for a minute or so. You can add at least a tablespoon of carrier oil and make a balm.

5. Digestive Soothing Mixture

This mixture works well as a vaporization mix that will leave the room feeling very atmospheric helping you to overcome your digestive problems.

Ingredients:

- 4 drops of rosewood essential oil

- 4 drops of ginger essential oil

- 2 drops of marjoram essential oil

Directions:

Add all of the ingredients into a small dark vial. Roll the vial around in your palm to mix oils. Inhale the oils for a minute or so. You can add at least a tablespoon of carrier oil and make a balm.

6. Immune Support Mixture

This wonderful mixture will help to support your immune system.

Ingredients:

- 4 drops of rosewood essential oil

- 4 drops of Frankincense essential oil

Directions:

Add all of the ingredients into a small dark vial. Roll the vial around in your palm to mix oils. Inhale the oils for a minute or so. You can add at least a tablespoon of carrier oil and make a balm.

7. Citrus System Refresher Blend

This blend will be like a cleanse that you can use year round to detox your system.

Ingredients:

- 20 drops of grapefruit essential oil

- 8 drops of lemon essential oil

- 1 tablespoon of sea salt

- 2 drops of Ylang Ylang essential oil

Directions:

Add all of the ingredients into a small dark vial. Roll the vial around in your palm to mix oils. Inhale the oils for a minute or so. You can add at least a tablespoon of carrier oil and make a balm.

8. Minty Relief

Using this mixture will help you to less likely suffer from acid reflux and help with digestive problems.

Ingredients:

- 4 drops of spearmint essential oil

- 5 drops of peppermint essential oil

- 4 drops of Ylang Ylang essential oil

- 1 tablespoon of sea salt

Directions:

Keep this mixture in a vaporizer in your dining area and it will help your loved ones to have a pleasant digestive process.

9. Healthier Skin Blend

This special blend will help deal with mental well-being, skin problems, menstrual cramps and detoxing all at the same time. Works well for those that aer finding life stressful.

Ingredients:

- 2 drops of grapefruit essential oil

- 4 drops of Bergamot essential oil

- 4 drops of Blood Orange essential oil

- 4 drops of Ylang Ylang essential oil

- 4 drops of Patchouli essential oil

Directions:

Add all of the ingredients into a small dark vial. Roll the vial around in your palm to mix oils. Inhale the oils for a minute or so. You can add at least a tablespoon of carrier cream to make cream to add to forehead to help relieve stress and create calm.

10. Grapefruit Detox Mix

This mix is great for helping to detox your skin, you can use this mix with any floral oil to have a great recipe for detoxing skin.

Ingredients:

- 6 drops of grapefruit essential oil

- 2 drops of jasmine essential oil

- 2 drops of clary sage essential oil

- at least one tablespoon of floral oil of your choice

Directions:

Add all of the ingredients into a small dark vial. Roll the vial around in your palm to mix oils. Inhale the oils for a minute or so. You can add at least a tablespoon of floral oil.

Conclusion

I hope that you and your loved ones will gain the many benefits attached to using essential oils to help you treat many common ailments. You are going to love using essential oils that are not filled with all kinds of synthetic ingredients and chemicals, but instead they are pure and natural with great remedies for many different ailments. A friend of mine introduced me into the world of essential oils about 30+ years ago, I can tell you that I am so glad she did. I still use them myself in my daily life today. I eventually expanded into growing many of my own medicinal plants in my garden. Of course you will decide what path you choose to go down with your essential oils whether you will buy them ready-made or decide at some point to make your own. I still buy most of my essential oils from my local health food store. It does take a lot of time and effort and plants to make your own oils at home. Whatever approach you decide to take I know you will be glad that you introduced essential oils into your everyday life!

I just wanted to thank you once again for downloading my book, I cannot express to you how grateful I truly am for this. I would love to read a review of my book written by you on Amazon. Take care, and happy life when you begin to reap the benefits of your essential oils!